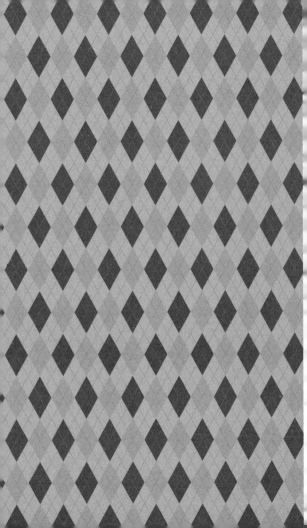

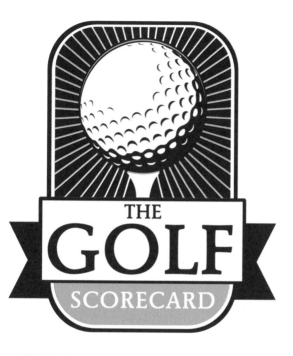

MASTER YOUR STATS

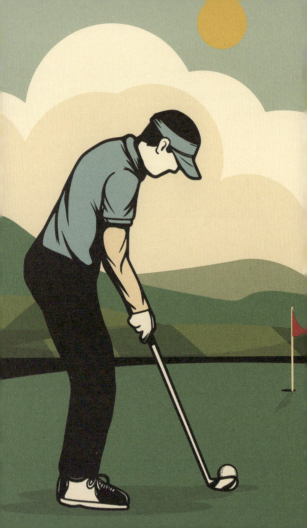

HOW TO USE YOUR GOLF GUIDE

RECORD PRACTICE TIME, SCORES, AND STATS

MY GOALS
Log your practice goals by writing down what you want to achieve and when you want to achieve each goal. For each quarter, define up to four goals with training ideas and tips for each. As you work toward your goals, record your progress and reflect on what went well and what can be improved.

PRACTICE LOG
The Practice Log tracks practice sessions over time to create repeated patterns for successful improvement. In this section, record up to fifty-two practice sessions with twenty drills per session—seventeen standard drills and room to add three unique drills that align with your personal goals.

First, create a training schedule by listing the drills or clubs to practice. Each drill should be accompanied by a **Distance Goal** or custom objective. Once practice begins, log the **Minutes Practiced**, **# of Balls Shot**, and **Shots Made** for each drill. To track your **Success Ratio**, divide the **Shots Made** by **# of Balls Shot**. After the session is finished, note your observations on what went well and what can be improved. Outline up to three drills to practice for your next session.

GAME SCORE AND STATS
Track and review scores, stats, and overall experience for up to eleven rounds of golf. Log standard data from your scorecard, including par, handicap, and score. Identify potential weaknesses and pay attention to trends in your stats that might need extra attention in practice. Understand your performance more accurately by logging advanced data and breaking down the front nine and back nine scores. In this section, log:

Fairways Hit and Club (Tee Shot): Number of fairways hit from your tee shot. Make sure to record the club used to better understand how your tee box game is affecting your overall game.

Green in Regulation (GIR): Eventually calculated as a percent, a green in regulation is recorded as "hit" if the birdie stroke on the hole is hit from the green. For each hole, log this as a 1 or 0 before adding up your totals. For more details, turn to the official PGA Tour rules and definitions: "If any portion of the ball is touching the putting surface after the GIR stroke" or the first stroke on a par-3, second stroke on a par-4, or third stroke on a par-5. Track this statistic over time; the percentage should increase as your game improves (which you will have the opportunity to log later in the journal).

Successful Scramble: Number of times you miss the green in regulation, but still make par or better. This measures your long game, as well as your resilience and mental fortitude.

Putts Per Round (PPR): Simply log the number of putts you had for each round. Calculate your putting average by dividing the number of putts taken by the number of holes played. This is a key indicator of a player's putting performance, but it's important to contextualize this statistic within the scope of all other data.

TOTALS

At the end of each round, compare rounds and track improvement over time by compiling your totals. Together with the standard summary, you can also log:

Driving ACC %: The percentage of time a tee shot comes to rest in the fairway (regardless of club). Divide the number of fairways hit by the number of attempts to calculate your percentage.

GIR %: Divide your green in regulation hit total by the total number of holes played. Although it's rarely common for amateur players to achieve a GIR, your percentage should increase over time and with practice drills.

Scramble %: Divide the number of successful scrambles by the total number of missed greens. The missed greens total is calculated by counting the number of greenside shots that missed the green. This statistic will help you understand your short game performance.

Average Putts: Divide the sum of your total putts by the number of holes played. Bringing this number down will have a significant impact on your scores. Aim to reduce your number of putts to three in each game.

Make sure to rate and rank each course you play. It's important to track your statistics to take your golf game to the next level. Over time, you'll practice more efficiently and improve your weaknesses. Set goals that motivate you, track your improvement, and, most importantly, have fun!

CALENDAR

Use the calendar to record your frequency of practice or play over one year. Strong golf performance is based on patience, precision, and focus. Tracking your practice and game days will keep front-of-mind important information, such as which holes you regularly score well on, which clubs you hit most accurately with, or which shots you struggle with. More data allows you to make informed, smart decisions more accurately during each round of golf, so it is vital to record each practice session—no matter how long or short. By consistently measuring how often you hit the links, you can set realistic performance goals and celebrate achieving them.

MY GOALS

QUARTER: _____ **YEAR:** _____

PLAN AND TIMELINE: _____
_____

GOAL #1

PLAN	PROGRESS	TIMELINE

GOAL #2

PLAN	PROGRESS	TIMELINE

GOAL #3

PLAN	PROGRESS	TIMELINE

GOAL #4

PLAN	PROGRESS	TIMELINE

MY GOALS

QUARTER: _____ **YEAR:** _____

PLAN AND TIMELINE: _____
_____

GOAL #1

PLAN	PROGRESS	TIMELINE

GOAL #2

PLAN	PROGRESS	TIMELINE

GOAL #3

PLAN	PROGRESS	TIMELINE

GOAL #4

PLAN	PROGRESS	TIMELINE

MY GOALS

QUARTER: _____ **YEAR:** _____

PLAN AND TIMELINE: _____
_____

GOAL #1

PLAN	PROGRESS	TIMELINE

GOAL #2

PLAN	PROGRESS	TIMELINE

GOAL #3

PLAN	PROGRESS	TIMELINE

GOAL #4

PLAN	PROGRESS	TIMELINE

MY GOALS

QUARTER: _____ **YEAR:** _____

PLAN AND TIMELINE: _____

GOAL #1

PLAN	PROGRESS	TIMELINE

GOAL #2

PLAN	PROGRESS	TIMELINE

GOAL #3

PLAN	PROGRESS	TIMELINE

GOAL #4

PLAN	PROGRESS	TIMELINE

PRACTICE LOG

SESSION OVERVIEW: DATE: _____ **LOCATION:** _____

START: _____ **END:** _____ S M T W T F S

CLUB/SHOT	DISTANCE GOAL	MINUTES PRACTICED	# OF BALLS	SHOTS MADE	SUCCESS RATIO
WARM UP					
PUTT					
PUTT					
PUTT					
PUTT					
9 IRON					
8 IRON					
7 IRON					
6 IRON					
5 IRON					
4 IRON					
3 IRON					
HYBRID					
DRIVER					
CHIPPING					
PITCHING					
OUT OF BUNKER					
TOTAL					

FAVORITE MOMENTS _____

AREAS OF IMPROVEMENT _____

TOP 3 DRILLS TO PRACTICE

1 _____

2 _____

3 _____

PRACTICE LOG

START: _____ END: _____ S M T W T F S

CLUB/SHOT	DISTANCE GOAL	MINUTES PRACTICED	# OF BALLS	SHOTS MADE	SUCCESS RATIO
WARM UP					
PUTT					
PUTT					
PUTT					
PUTT					
9 IRON					
8 IRON					
7 IRON					
6 IRON					
5 IRON					
4 IRON					
3 IRON					
HYBRID					
DRIVER					
CHIPPING					
PITCHING					
OUT OF BUNKER					
TOTAL					

FAVORITE MOMENTS _____

_____

AREAS OF IMPROVEMENT _____

TOP 3 DRILLS TO PRACTICE

1. _____

2. _____

3. _____

PRACTICE LOG

SESSION OVERVIEW: DATE: _____ **LOCATION:** _____

START: _____ **END:** _____ S M T W T F S

CLUB/SHOT	DISTANCE GOAL	MINUTES PRACTICED	# OF BALLS	SHOTS MADE	SUCCESS RATIO
WARM UP					
PUTT					
PUTT					
PUTT					
PUTT					
9 IRON					
8 IRON					
7 IRON					
6 IRON					
5 IRON					
4 IRON					
3 IRON					
HYBRID					
DRIVER					
CHIPPING					
PITCHING					
OUT OF BUNKER					
TOTAL					

FAVORITE MOMENTS _____

_____

_____

AREAS OF IMPROVEMENT _____

_____

_____

TOP 3 DRILLS TO PRACTICE

1 _____

2 _____

3 _____

PRACTICE LOG

START: _____ END: _____ S M T W T F S

CLUB/SHOT	DISTANCE GOAL	MINUTES PRACTICED	# OF BALLS	SHOTS MADE	SUCCESS RATIO
WARM UP					
PUTT					
PUTT					
PUTT					
PUTT					
9 IRON					
8 IRON					
7 IRON					
6 IRON					
5 IRON					
4 IRON					
3 IRON					
HYBRID					
DRIVER					
CHIPPING					
PITCHING					
OUT OF BUNKER					
TOTAL					

FAVORITE MOMENTS _____

_____

_____

AREAS OF IMPROVEMENT _____

TOP 3 DRILLS TO PRACTICE

1 _____

2 _____

3 _____

PRACTICE LOG

SESSION OVERVIEW: DATE: _____ **LOCATION:** _____

START: _____ **END:** _____ S M T W T F S

CLUB/SHOT	DISTANCE GOAL	MINUTES PRACTICED	# OF BALLS	SHOTS MADE	SUCCESS RATIO
WARM UP					
PUTT					
PUTT					
PUTT					
PUTT					
9 IRON					
8 IRON					
7 IRON					
6 IRON					
5 IRON					
4 IRON					
3 IRON					
HYBRID					
DRIVER					
CHIPPING					
PITCHING					
OUT OF BUNKER					
TOTAL					

FAVORITE MOMENTS _____

AREAS OF IMPROVEMENT _____

TOP 3 DRILLS TO PRACTICE

1 _____

2 _____

3 _____

PRACTICE LOG

START: _____ **END:** _____   S   M   T   W   T   F   S

CLUB/SHOT	DISTANCE GOAL	MINUTES PRACTICED	# OF BALLS	SHOTS MADE	SUCCESS RATIO
WARM UP					
PUTT					
PUTT					
PUTT					
PUTT					
9 IRON					
8 IRON					
7 IRON					
6 IRON					
5 IRON					
4 IRON					
3 IRON					
HYBRID					
DRIVER					
CHIPPING					
PITCHING					
OUT OF BUNKER					
TOTAL					

FAVORITE MOMENTS _____

AREAS OF IMPROVEMENT _____

TOP 3 DRILLS TO PRACTICE

1 _____

2 _____

3 _____

PRACTICE LOG

SESSION OVERVIEW: DATE: _____ **LOCATION:** _____

START: _____ **END:** _____ S M T W T F S

CLUB/SHOT	DISTANCE GOAL	MINUTES PRACTICED	# OF BALLS	SHOTS MADE	SUCCESS RATIO
WARM UP					
PUTT					
PUTT					
PUTT					
PUTT					
9 IRON					
8 IRON					
7 IRON					
6 IRON					
5 IRON					
4 IRON					
3 IRON					
HYBRID					
DRIVER					
CHIPPING					
PITCHING					
OUT OF BUNKER					
TOTAL					

FAVORITE MOMENTS _____

_____

_____

AREAS OF IMPROVEMENT _____

_____

_____

TOP 3 DRILLS TO PRACTICE

1 _____

2 _____

3 _____

PRACTICE LOG

START: _____ **END:** _____   S   M   T   W   T   F   S

CLUB/SHOT	DISTANCE GOAL	MINUTES PRACTICED	# OF BALLS	SHOTS MADE	SUCCESS RATIO
WARM UP					
PUTT					
PUTT					
PUTT					
PUTT					
9 IRON					
8 IRON					
7 IRON					
6 IRON					
5 IRON					
4 IRON					
3 IRON					
HYBRID					
DRIVER					
CHIPPING					
PITCHING					
OUT OF BUNKER					
TOTAL					

FAVORITE MOMENTS _____

_____

_____

AREAS OF IMPROVEMENT _____

_____

TOP 3 DRILLS TO PRACTICE

1. _____

2. _____

3. _____

PRACTICE LOG

SESSION OVERVIEW: DATE: _____ **LOCATION:** _____

START: _____ **END:** _____ S M T W T F S

CLUB/SHOT	DISTANCE GOAL	MINUTES PRACTICED	# OF BALLS	SHOTS MADE	SUCCESS RATIO
WARM UP					
PUTT					
PUTT					
PUTT					
PUTT					
9 IRON					
8 IRON					
7 IRON					
6 IRON					
5 IRON					
4 IRON					
3 IRON					
HYBRID					
DRIVER					
CHIPPING					
PITCHING					
OUT OF BUNKER					
TOTAL					

FAVORITE MOMENTS _____
_____
_____

AREAS OF IMPROVEMENT _____
_____
_____

TOP 3 DRILLS TO PRACTICE

1 _____

2 _____

3 _____

PRACTICE LOG

START: _____ **END:** _____ S M T W T F S

CLUB/SHOT	DISTANCE GOAL	MINUTES PRACTICED	# OF BALLS	SHOTS MADE	SUCCESS RATIO
WARM UP					
PUTT					
PUTT					
PUTT					
PUTT					
9 IRON					
8 IRON					
7 IRON					
6 IRON					
5 IRON					
4 IRON					
3 IRON					
HYBRID					
DRIVER					
CHIPPING					
PITCHING					
OUT OF BUNKER					
TOTAL					

FAVORITE MOMENTS _____

_____

_____

AREAS OF IMPROVEMENT _____

_____

TOP 3 DRILLS TO PRACTICE

1 _____

2 _____

3 _____

PRACTICE LOG

SESSION OVERVIEW: DATE: _____ **LOCATION:** _____

START: _____ **END:** _____ S M T W T F S

CLUB/SHOT	DISTANCE GOAL	MINUTES PRACTICED	# OF BALLS	SHOTS MADE	SUCCESS RATIO
WARM UP					
PUTT					
PUTT					
PUTT					
PUTT					
9 IRON					
8 IRON					
7 IRON					
6 IRON					
5 IRON					
4 IRON					
3 IRON					
HYBRID					
DRIVER					
CHIPPING					
PITCHING					
OUT OF BUNKER					
TOTAL					

FAVORITE MOMENTS _____
_____
_____

AREAS OF IMPROVEMENT _____
_____
_____

TOP 3 DRILLS TO PRACTICE

1 _____

2 _____

3 _____

PRACTICE LOG

START: _____ **END:** _____ S M T W T F S

CLUB/SHOT	DISTANCE GOAL	MINUTES PRACTICED	# OF BALLS	SHOTS MADE	SUCCESS RATIO
WARM UP					
PUTT					
PUTT					
PUTT					
PUTT					
9 IRON					
8 IRON					
7 IRON					
6 IRON					
5 IRON					
4 IRON					
3 IRON					
HYBRID					
DRIVER					
CHIPPING					
PITCHING					
OUT OF BUNKER					
TOTAL					

FAVORITE MOMENTS _____

_____

AREAS OF IMPROVEMENT _____

TOP 3 DRILLS TO PRACTICE

1 _____

2 _____

3 _____

PRACTICE LOG

SESSION OVERVIEW: DATE: _____ **LOCATION:** _____

START: _____ **END:** _____ S M T W T F S

CLUB/SHOT	DISTANCE GOAL	MINUTES PRACTICED	# OF BALLS	SHOTS MADE	SUCCESS RATIO
WARM UP					
PUTT					
PUTT					
PUTT					
PUTT					
9 IRON					
8 IRON					
7 IRON					
6 IRON					
5 IRON					
4 IRON					
3 IRON					
HYBRID					
DRIVER					
CHIPPING					
PITCHING					
OUT OF BUNKER					
TOTAL					

FAVORITE MOMENTS _____
_____
_____

AREAS OF IMPROVEMENT _____
_____
_____

TOP 3 DRILLS TO PRACTICE

1 _____

2 _____

3 _____

PRACTICE LOG

START: _____ **END:** _____ S M T W T F S

CLUB/SHOT	DISTANCE GOAL	MINUTES PRACTICED	# OF BALLS	SHOTS MADE	SUCCESS RATIO
WARM UP					
PUTT					
PUTT					
PUTT					
PUTT					
9 IRON					
8 IRON					
7 IRON					
6 IRON					
5 IRON					
4 IRON					
3 IRON					
HYBRID					
DRIVER					
CHIPPING					
PITCHING					
OUT OF BUNKER					
TOTAL					

FAVORITE MOMENTS _____

_____

AREAS OF IMPROVEMENT _____

_____

TOP 3 DRILLS TO PRACTICE

1 _____

2 _____

3 _____

PRACTICE LOG

SESSION OVERVIEW: DATE: _____ **LOCATION:** _____

START: _____ **END:** _____ S M T W T F S

CLUB/SHOT	DISTANCE GOAL	MINUTES PRACTICED	# OF BALLS	SHOTS MADE	SUCCESS RATIO
WARM UP					
PUTT					
PUTT					
PUTT					
PUTT					
9 IRON					
8 IRON					
7 IRON					
6 IRON					
5 IRON					
4 IRON					
3 IRON					
HYBRID					
DRIVER					
CHIPPING					
PITCHING					
OUT OF BUNKER					
TOTAL					

FAVORITE MOMENTS _____

_____

_____

AREAS OF IMPROVEMENT _____

_____

_____

TOP 3 DRILLS TO PRACTICE

1 _____

_____

2 _____

_____

3 _____

PRACTICE LOG

START: _____ **END:** _____ S M T W T F S

CLUB/SHOT	DISTANCE GOAL	MINUTES PRACTICED	# OF BALLS	SHOTS MADE	SUCCESS RATIO
WARM UP					
PUTT					
PUTT					
PUTT					
PUTT					
9 IRON					
8 IRON					
7 IRON					
6 IRON					
5 IRON					
4 IRON					
3 IRON					
HYBRID					
DRIVER					
CHIPPING					
PITCHING					
OUT OF BUNKER					
TOTAL					

FAVORITE MOMENTS _____

_____

_____

AREAS OF IMPROVEMENT _____

TOP 3 DRILLS TO PRACTICE

1 _____

2 _____

3 _____

PRACTICE LOG

SESSION OVERVIEW: DATE: _____ **LOCATION:** _____

START: _____ **END:** _____ S M T W T F S

CLUB/SHOT	DISTANCE GOAL	MINUTES PRACTICED	# OF BALLS	SHOTS MADE	SUCCESS RATIO
WARM UP					
PUTT					
PUTT					
PUTT					
PUTT					
9 IRON					
8 IRON					
7 IRON					
6 IRON					
5 IRON					
4 IRON					
3 IRON					
HYBRID					
DRIVER					
CHIPPING					
PITCHING					
OUT OF BUNKER					
TOTAL					

FAVORITE MOMENTS _____

_____

_____

AREAS OF IMPROVEMENT _____

_____

_____

TOP 3 DRILLS TO PRACTICE

1 _____

2 _____

3 _____

PRACTICE LOG

START: _____ END: _____ S M T W T F S

CLUB/SHOT	DISTANCE GOAL	MINUTES PRACTICED	# OF BALLS	SHOTS MADE	SUCCESS RATIO
WARM UP					
PUTT					
PUTT					
PUTT					
PUTT					
9 IRON					
8 IRON					
7 IRON					
6 IRON					
5 IRON					
4 IRON					
3 IRON					
HYBRID					
DRIVER					
CHIPPING					
PITCHING					
OUT OF BUNKER					
TOTAL					

FAVORITE MOMENTS _____

AREAS OF IMPROVEMENT _____

TOP 3 DRILLS TO PRACTICE

1 _____

2 _____

3 _____

PRACTICE LOG

SESSION OVERVIEW: DATE: _____ **LOCATION:** _____

START: _____ **END:** _____ S M T W T F S

CLUB/SHOT	DISTANCE GOAL	MINUTES PRACTICED	# OF BALLS	SHOTS MADE	SUCCESS RATIO
WARM UP					
PUTT					
PUTT					
PUTT					
PUTT					
9 IRON					
8 IRON					
7 IRON					
6 IRON					
5 IRON					
4 IRON					
3 IRON					
HYBRID					
DRIVER					
CHIPPING					
PITCHING					
OUT OF BUNKER					
TOTAL					

FAVORITE MOMENTS _____
_____
_____

AREAS OF IMPROVEMENT _____
_____
_____

TOP 3 DRILLS TO PRACTICE

1 _____
_____
2 _____
_____
3 _____

PRACTICE LOG

START: _____ **END:** _____ S M T W T F S

CLUB/SHOT	DISTANCE GOAL	MINUTES PRACTICED	# OF BALLS	SHOTS MADE	SUCCESS RATIO
WARM UP					
PUTT					
PUTT					
PUTT					
PUTT					
9 IRON					
8 IRON					
7 IRON					
6 IRON					
5 IRON					
4 IRON					
3 IRON					
HYBRID					
DRIVER					
CHIPPING					
PITCHING					
OUT OF BUNKER					
TOTAL					

FAVORITE MOMENTS _____

AREAS OF IMPROVEMENT _____

TOP 3 DRILLS TO PRACTICE

1 _____

2 _____

3 _____

PRACTICE LOG

SESSION OVERVIEW: DATE: _____ **LOCATION:** _____

START: _____ **END:** _____ S M T W T F S

CLUB/SHOT	DISTANCE GOAL	MINUTES PRACTICED	# OF BALLS	SHOTS MADE	SUCCESS RATIO
WARM UP					
PUTT					
PUTT					
PUTT					
PUTT					
9 IRON					
8 IRON					
7 IRON					
6 IRON					
5 IRON					
4 IRON					
3 IRON					
HYBRID					
DRIVER					
CHIPPING					
PITCHING					
OUT OF BUNKER					
TOTAL					

FAVORITE MOMENTS _____
_____
_____

AREAS OF IMPROVEMENT _____
_____
_____

TOP 3 DRILLS TO PRACTICE

1 _____

2 _____

3 _____

PRACTICE LOG

START: _____ **END:** _____ S M T W T F S

CLUB/SHOT	DISTANCE GOAL	MINUTES PRACTICED	# OF BALLS	SHOTS MADE	SUCCESS RATIO
WARM UP					
PUTT					
PUTT					
PUTT					
PUTT					
9 IRON					
8 IRON					
7 IRON					
6 IRON					
5 IRON					
4 IRON					
3 IRON					
HYBRID					
DRIVER					
CHIPPING					
PITCHING					
OUT OF BUNKER					
TOTAL					

FAVORITE MOMENTS _____

_____

_____

AREAS OF IMPROVEMENT _____

TOP 3 DRILLS TO PRACTICE

1 _____

2 _____

3 _____

PRACTICE LOG

SESSION OVERVIEW: DATE: _____ **LOCATION:** _____

START: _____ **END:** _____ S M T W T F S

CLUB/SHOT	DISTANCE GOAL	MINUTES PRACTICED	# OF BALLS	SHOTS MADE	SUCCESS RATIO
WARM UP					
PUTT					
PUTT					
PUTT					
PUTT					
9 IRON					
8 IRON					
7 IRON					
6 IRON					
5 IRON					
4 IRON					
3 IRON					
HYBRID					
DRIVER					
CHIPPING					
PITCHING					
OUT OF BUNKER					
TOTAL					

FAVORITE MOMENTS _____

AREAS OF IMPROVEMENT _____

TOP 3 DRILLS TO PRACTICE

1 _____

2 _____

3 _____

PRACTICE LOG

START: _____ **END:** _____ S M T W T F S

CLUB/SHOT	DISTANCE GOAL	MINUTES PRACTICED	# OF BALLS	SHOTS MADE	SUCCESS RATIO
WARM UP					
PUTT					
PUTT					
PUTT					
PUTT					
9 IRON					
8 IRON					
7 IRON					
6 IRON					
5 IRON					
4 IRON					
3 IRON					
HYBRID					
DRIVER					
CHIPPING					
PITCHING					
OUT OF BUNKER					
TOTAL					

FAVORITE MOMENTS _____

AREAS OF IMPROVEMENT _____

TOP 3 DRILLS TO PRACTICE

1 _____

2 _____

3 _____

PRACTICE LOG

SESSION OVERVIEW: DATE: _____ **LOCATION:** _____

START: _____ **END:** _____   S   M   T   W   T   F   S

CLUB/SHOT	DISTANCE GOAL	MINUTES PRACTICED	# OF BALLS	SHOTS MADE	SUCCESS RATIO
WARM UP					
PUTT					
PUTT					
PUTT					
PUTT					
9 IRON					
8 IRON					
7 IRON					
6 IRON					
5 IRON					
4 IRON					
3 IRON					
HYBRID					
DRIVER					
CHIPPING					
PITCHING					
OUT OF BUNKER					
TOTAL					

FAVORITE MOMENTS _____

AREAS OF IMPROVEMENT _____

TOP 3 DRILLS TO PRACTICE

1 _____

2 _____

3 _____

PRACTICE LOG

START: _____ END: _____ S M T W T F S

CLUB/SHOT	DISTANCE GOAL	MINUTES PRACTICED	# OF BALLS	SHOTS MADE	SUCCESS RATIO
WARM UP					
PUTT					
PUTT					
PUTT					
PUTT					
9 IRON					
8 IRON					
7 IRON					
6 IRON					
5 IRON					
4 IRON					
3 IRON					
HYBRID					
DRIVER					
CHIPPING					
PITCHING					
OUT OF BUNKER					
TOTAL					

FAVORITE MOMENTS _____

_____

_____

AREAS OF IMPROVEMENT _____

_____

TOP 3 DRILLS TO PRACTICE

1 _____

2 _____

3 _____

PRACTICE LOG

SESSION OVERVIEW: DATE: _____ **LOCATION:** _____

START: _____ **END:** _____ S M T W T F S

CLUB/SHOT	DISTANCE GOAL	MINUTES PRACTICED	# OF BALLS	SHOTS MADE	SUCCESS RATIO
WARM UP					
PUTT					
PUTT					
PUTT					
PUTT					
9 IRON					
8 IRON					
7 IRON					
6 IRON					
5 IRON					
4 IRON					
3 IRON					
HYBRID					
DRIVER					
CHIPPING					
PITCHING					
OUT OF BUNKER					
TOTAL					

FAVORITE MOMENTS _____
_____
_____

AREAS OF IMPROVEMENT _____
_____
_____

TOP 3 DRILLS TO PRACTICE

1 _____

2 _____

3 _____

PRACTICE LOG

START: _____ **END:** _____ S M T W T F S

CLUB/SHOT	DISTANCE GOAL	MINUTES PRACTICED	# OF BALLS	SHOTS MADE	SUCCESS RATIO
WARM UP					
PUTT					
PUTT					
PUTT					
PUTT					
9 IRON					
8 IRON					
7 IRON					
6 IRON					
5 IRON					
4 IRON					
3 IRON					
HYBRID					
DRIVER					
CHIPPING					
PITCHING					
OUT OF BUNKER					
TOTAL					

FAVORITE MOMENTS _____

AREAS OF IMPROVEMENT _____

TOP 3 DRILLS TO PRACTICE

1 _____

2 _____

3 _____

PRACTICE LOG

SESSION OVERVIEW: DATE: _____ **LOCATION:** _____

START: _____ **END:** _____ S M T W T F S

CLUB/SHOT	DISTANCE GOAL	MINUTES PRACTICED	# OF BALLS	SHOTS MADE	SUCCESS RATIO
WARM UP					
PUTT					
PUTT					
PUTT					
PUTT					
9 IRON					
8 IRON					
7 IRON					
6 IRON					
5 IRON					
4 IRON					
3 IRON					
HYBRID					
DRIVER					
CHIPPING					
PITCHING					
OUT OF BUNKER					
TOTAL					

FAVORITE MOMENTS _____
_____
_____

AREAS OF IMPROVEMENT _____
_____

TOP 3 DRILLS TO PRACTICE

1 _____

2 _____

3 _____

PRACTICE LOG

START: _____ END: _____   S M T W T F S

CLUB/SHOT	DISTANCE GOAL	MINUTES PRACTICED	# OF BALLS	SHOTS MADE	SUCCESS RATIO
WARM UP					
PUTT					
PUTT					
PUTT					
PUTT					
9 IRON					
8 IRON					
7 IRON					
6 IRON					
5 IRON					
4 IRON					
3 IRON					
HYBRID					
DRIVER					
CHIPPING					
PITCHING					
OUT OF BUNKER					
TOTAL					

FAVORITE MOMENTS _____

AREAS OF IMPROVEMENT _____

TOP 3 DRILLS TO PRACTICE

1 _____

2 _____

3 _____

PRACTICE LOG

SESSION OVERVIEW: DATE: _____ **LOCATION:** _____

START: _____ **END:** _____ S M T W T F S

CLUB/SHOT	DISTANCE GOAL	MINUTES PRACTICED	# OF BALLS	SHOTS MADE	SUCCESS RATIO
WARM UP					
PUTT					
PUTT					
PUTT					
PUTT					
9 IRON					
8 IRON					
7 IRON					
6 IRON					
5 IRON					
4 IRON					
3 IRON					
HYBRID					
DRIVER					
CHIPPING					
PITCHING					
OUT OF BUNKER					
TOTAL					

FAVORITE MOMENTS _____

AREAS OF IMPROVEMENT _____

TOP 3 DRILLS TO PRACTICE

1 _____

2 _____

3 _____

PRACTICE LOG

START: _____ **END:** _____ S M T W T F S

CLUB/SHOT	DISTANCE GOAL	MINUTES PRACTICED	# OF BALLS	SHOTS MADE	SUCCESS RATIO
WARM UP					
PUTT					
PUTT					
PUTT					
PUTT					
9 IRON					
8 IRON					
7 IRON					
6 IRON					
5 IRON					
4 IRON					
3 IRON					
HYBRID					
DRIVER					
CHIPPING					
PITCHING					
OUT OF BUNKER					
TOTAL					

FAVORITE MOMENTS _____

AREAS OF IMPROVEMENT _____

TOP 3 DRILLS TO PRACTICE

1 _____

2 _____

3 _____

PRACTICE LOG

SESSION OVERVIEW: DATE: _____ **LOCATION:** _____

START: _____ **END:** _____ S M T W T F S

CLUB/SHOT	DISTANCE GOAL	MINUTES PRACTICED	# OF BALLS	SHOTS MADE	SUCCESS RATIO
WARM UP					
PUTT					
PUTT					
PUTT					
PUTT					
9 IRON					
8 IRON					
7 IRON					
6 IRON					
5 IRON					
4 IRON					
3 IRON					
HYBRID					
DRIVER					
CHIPPING					
PITCHING					
OUT OF BUNKER					
TOTAL					

FAVORITE MOMENTS _____

AREAS OF IMPROVEMENT _____

TOP 3 DRILLS TO PRACTICE

1 _____

2 _____

3 _____

PRACTICE LOG

START: _____ END: _____   S   M   T   W   T   F   S

CLUB/SHOT	DISTANCE GOAL	MINUTES PRACTICED	# OF BALLS	SHOTS MADE	SUCCESS RATIO
WARM UP					
PUTT					
PUTT					
PUTT					
PUTT					
9 IRON					
8 IRON					
7 IRON					
6 IRON					
5 IRON					
4 IRON					
3 IRON					
HYBRID					
DRIVER					
CHIPPING					
PITCHING					
OUT OF BUNKER					
TOTAL					

FAVORITE MOMENTS _____

_____

_____

AREAS OF IMPROVEMENT _____

_____

TOP 3 DRILLS TO PRACTICE

1 _____

2 _____

3 _____

PRACTICE LOG

SESSION OVERVIEW: DATE: _____ **LOCATION:** _____

START: _____ **END:** _____ S M T W T F S

CLUB/SHOT	DISTANCE GOAL	MINUTES PRACTICED	# OF BALLS	SHOTS MADE	SUCCESS RATIO
WARM UP					
PUTT					
PUTT					
PUTT					
PUTT					
9 IRON					
8 IRON					
7 IRON					
6 IRON					
5 IRON					
4 IRON					
3 IRON					
HYBRID					
DRIVER					
CHIPPING					
PITCHING					
OUT OF BUNKER					
TOTAL					

FAVORITE MOMENTS _____
_____
_____

AREAS OF IMPROVEMENT _____
_____
_____

TOP 3 DRILLS TO PRACTICE

1 _____
_____

2 _____
_____

3 _____
_____

PRACTICE LOG

START: _____ **END:** _____ S M T W T F S

CLUB/SHOT	DISTANCE GOAL	MINUTES PRACTICED	# OF BALLS	SHOTS MADE	SUCCESS RATIO
WARM UP					
PUTT					
PUTT					
PUTT					
PUTT					
9 IRON					
8 IRON					
7 IRON					
6 IRON					
5 IRON					
4 IRON					
3 IRON					
HYBRID					
DRIVER					
CHIPPING					
PITCHING					
OUT OF BUNKER					
TOTAL					

FAVORITE MOMENTS _____

_____

_____

AREAS OF IMPROVEMENT _____

TOP 3 DRILLS TO PRACTICE

1 _____

2 _____

3 _____

PRACTICE LOG

SESSION OVERVIEW: DATE: _____ **LOCATION:** _____

START: _____ **END:** _____   S   M   T   W   T   F   S

CLUB/SHOT	DISTANCE GOAL	MINUTES PRACTICED	# OF BALLS	SHOTS MADE	SUCCESS RATIO
WARM UP					
PUTT					
PUTT					
PUTT					
PUTT					
9 IRON					
8 IRON					
7 IRON					
6 IRON					
5 IRON					
4 IRON					
3 IRON					
HYBRID					
DRIVER					
CHIPPING					
PITCHING					
OUT OF BUNKER					
TOTAL					

FAVORITE MOMENTS _____

_____

_____

AREAS OF IMPROVEMENT _____

_____

_____

TOP 3 DRILLS TO PRACTICE

1 _____

2 _____

3 _____

PRACTICE LOG

START: _____ **END:** _____ S M T W T F S

CLUB/SHOT	DISTANCE GOAL	MINUTES PRACTICED	# OF BALLS	SHOTS MADE	SUCCESS RATIO
WARM UP					
PUTT					
PUTT					
PUTT					
PUTT					
9 IRON					
8 IRON					
7 IRON					
6 IRON					
5 IRON					
4 IRON					
3 IRON					
HYBRID					
DRIVER					
CHIPPING					
PITCHING					
OUT OF BUNKER					
TOTAL					

FAVORITE MOMENTS _____

_____

_____

AREAS OF IMPROVEMENT _____

_____

TOP 3 DRILLS TO PRACTICE

1 _____

2 _____

3 _____

PRACTICE LOG

SESSION OVERVIEW: DATE: _____ **LOCATION:** _____

START: _____ **END:** _____ S M T W T F S

CLUB/SHOT	DISTANCE GOAL	MINUTES PRACTICED	# OF BALLS	SHOTS MADE	SUCCESS RATIO
WARM UP					
PUTT					
PUTT					
PUTT					
PUTT					
9 IRON					
8 IRON					
7 IRON					
6 IRON					
5 IRON					
4 IRON					
3 IRON					
HYBRID					
DRIVER					
CHIPPING					
PITCHING					
OUT OF BUNKER					
TOTAL					

FAVORITE MOMENTS _____
_____
_____

AREAS OF IMPROVEMENT _____
_____
_____

TOP 3 DRILLS TO PRACTICE

1 _____

2 _____

3 _____

PRACTICE LOG

START: _____ **END:** _____ S M T W T F S

CLUB/SHOT	DISTANCE GOAL	MINUTES PRACTICED	# OF BALLS	SHOTS MADE	SUCCESS RATIO
WARM UP					
PUTT					
PUTT					
PUTT					
PUTT					
9 IRON					
8 IRON					
7 IRON					
6 IRON					
5 IRON					
4 IRON					
3 IRON					
HYBRID					
DRIVER					
CHIPPING					
PITCHING					
OUT OF BUNKER					
TOTAL					

FAVORITE MOMENTS _____

_____

AREAS OF IMPROVEMENT _____

TOP 3 DRILLS TO PRACTICE

1 _____

2 _____

3 _____

PRACTICE LOG

SESSION OVERVIEW: DATE: _____ **LOCATION:** _____

START: _____ **END:** _____ S M T W T F S

CLUB/SHOT	DISTANCE GOAL	MINUTES PRACTICED	# OF BALLS	SHOTS MADE	SUCCESS RATIO
WARM UP					
PUTT					
PUTT					
PUTT					
PUTT					
9 IRON					
8 IRON					
7 IRON					
6 IRON					
5 IRON					
4 IRON					
3 IRON					
HYBRID					
DRIVER					
CHIPPING					
PITCHING					
OUT OF BUNKER					
TOTAL					

FAVORITE MOMENTS _____
_____
_____

AREAS OF IMPROVEMENT _____
_____
_____

TOP 3 DRILLS TO PRACTICE

1 _____

2 _____

3 _____

PRACTICE LOG

START: _____ **END:** _____ S M T W T F S

CLUB/SHOT	DISTANCE GOAL	MINUTES PRACTICED	# OF BALLS	SHOTS MADE	SUCCESS RATIO
WARM UP					
PUTT					
PUTT					
PUTT					
PUTT					
9 IRON					
8 IRON					
7 IRON					
6 IRON					
5 IRON					
4 IRON					
3 IRON					
HYBRID					
DRIVER					
CHIPPING					
PITCHING					
OUT OF BUNKER					
TOTAL					

FAVORITE MOMENTS _____

_____

_____

AREAS OF IMPROVEMENT _____

_____

TOP 3 DRILLS TO PRACTICE

1 _____

2 _____

3 _____

PRACTICE LOG

SESSION OVERVIEW: DATE: _____ **LOCATION:** _____

START: _____ **END:** _____ S M T W T F S

CLUB/SHOT	DISTANCE GOAL	MINUTES PRACTICED	# OF BALLS	SHOTS MADE	SUCCESS RATIO
WARM UP					
PUTT					
PUTT					
PUTT					
PUTT					
9 IRON					
8 IRON					
7 IRON					
6 IRON					
5 IRON					
4 IRON					
3 IRON					
HYBRID					
DRIVER					
CHIPPING					
PITCHING					
OUT OF BUNKER					
TOTAL					

FAVORITE MOMENTS _____
_____
_____

AREAS OF IMPROVEMENT _____
_____
_____

TOP 3 DRILLS TO PRACTICE

1 _____
_____
2 _____
_____
3 _____

PRACTICE LOG

START: _____ **END:** _____ S M T W T F S

CLUB/SHOT	DISTANCE GOAL	MINUTES PRACTICED	# OF BALLS	SHOTS MADE	SUCCESS RATIO
WARM UP					
PUTT					
PUTT					
PUTT					
PUTT					
9 IRON					
8 IRON					
7 IRON					
6 IRON					
5 IRON					
4 IRON					
3 IRON					
HYBRID					
DRIVER					
CHIPPING					
PITCHING					
OUT OF BUNKER					
TOTAL					

FAVORITE MOMENTS _____

AREAS OF IMPROVEMENT _____

TOP 3 DRILLS TO PRACTICE

1 _____

2 _____

3 _____

PRACTICE LOG

SESSION OVERVIEW: DATE: _____ **LOCATION:** _____

START: _____ **END:** _____ S M T W T F S

CLUB/SHOT	DISTANCE GOAL	MINUTES PRACTICED	# OF BALLS	SHOTS MADE	SUCCESS RATIO
WARM UP					
PUTT					
PUTT					
PUTT					
PUTT					
9 IRON					
8 IRON					
7 IRON					
6 IRON					
5 IRON					
4 IRON					
3 IRON					
HYBRID					
DRIVER					
CHIPPING					
PITCHING					
OUT OF BUNKER					
TOTAL					

FAVORITE MOMENTS _____

AREAS OF IMPROVEMENT _____

TOP 3 DRILLS TO PRACTICE

1 _____

2 _____

3 _____

PRACTICE LOG

START: _____ **END:** _____ S M T W T F S

CLUB/SHOT	DISTANCE GOAL	MINUTES PRACTICED	# OF BALLS	SHOTS MADE	SUCCESS RATIO
WARM UP					
PUTT					
PUTT					
PUTT					
PUTT					
9 IRON					
8 IRON					
7 IRON					
6 IRON					
5 IRON					
4 IRON					
3 IRON					
HYBRID					
DRIVER					
CHIPPING					
PITCHING					
OUT OF BUNKER					
TOTAL					

FAVORITE MOMENTS _____

AREAS OF IMPROVEMENT _____

TOP 3 DRILLS TO PRACTICE

1 _____

2 _____

3 _____

PRACTICE LOG

SESSION OVERVIEW: DATE: _____ **LOCATION:** _____

START: _____ **END:** _____ S M T W T F S

CLUB/SHOT	DISTANCE GOAL	MINUTES PRACTICED	# OF BALLS	SHOTS MADE	SUCCESS RATIO
WARM UP					
PUTT					
PUTT					
PUTT					
PUTT					
9 IRON					
8 IRON					
7 IRON					
6 IRON					
5 IRON					
4 IRON					
3 IRON					
HYBRID					
DRIVER					
CHIPPING					
PITCHING					
OUT OF BUNKER					
TOTAL					

FAVORITE MOMENTS _____

_____

_____

AREAS OF IMPROVEMENT _____

_____

_____

TOP 3 DRILLS TO PRACTICE

1 _____

2 _____

3 _____

PRACTICE LOG

START: _____ **END:** _____ S M T W T F S

CLUB/SHOT	DISTANCE GOAL	MINUTES PRACTICED	# OF BALLS	SHOTS MADE	SUCCESS RATIO
WARM UP					
PUTT					
PUTT					
PUTT					
PUTT					
9 IRON					
8 IRON					
7 IRON					
6 IRON					
5 IRON					
4 IRON					
3 IRON					
HYBRID					
DRIVER					
CHIPPING					
PITCHING					
OUT OF BUNKER					
TOTAL					

FAVORITE MOMENTS _____

_____

AREAS OF IMPROVEMENT _____

TOP 3 DRILLS TO PRACTICE

1 _____

2 _____

3 _____

PRACTICE LOG

SESSION OVERVIEW: DATE: _____ **LOCATION:** _____

START: _____ **END:** _____ S M T W T F S

CLUB/SHOT	DISTANCE GOAL	MINUTES PRACTICED	# OF BALLS	SHOTS MADE	SUCCESS RATIO
WARM UP					
PUTT					
PUTT					
PUTT					
PUTT					
9 IRON					
8 IRON					
7 IRON					
6 IRON					
5 IRON					
4 IRON					
3 IRON					
HYBRID					
DRIVER					
CHIPPING					
PITCHING					
OUT OF BUNKER					
TOTAL					

FAVORITE MOMENTS _____

AREAS OF IMPROVEMENT _____

TOP 3 DRILLS TO PRACTICE

1 _____

2 _____

3 _____

PRACTICE LOG

_____   _____

START: _____ END: _____   S M T W T F S

CLUB/SHOT	DISTANCE GOAL	MINUTES PRACTICED	# OF BALLS	SHOTS MADE	SUCCESS RATIO
WARM UP					
PUTT					
PUTT					
PUTT					
PUTT					
9 IRON					
8 IRON					
7 IRON					
6 IRON					
5 IRON					
4 IRON					
3 IRON					
HYBRID					
DRIVER					
CHIPPING					
PITCHING					
OUT OF BUNKER					
TOTAL					

FAVORITE MOMENTS _____

_____

_____

AREAS OF IMPROVEMENT _____

_____

TOP 3 DRILLS TO PRACTICE

1 _____

2 _____

3 _____

PRACTICE LOG

SESSION OVERVIEW: DATE: _____ **LOCATION:** _____

START: _____ **END:** _____ S M T W T F S

CLUB/SHOT	DISTANCE GOAL	MINUTES PRACTICED	# OF BALLS	SHOTS MADE	SUCCESS RATIO
WARM UP					
PUTT					
PUTT					
PUTT					
PUTT					
9 IRON					
8 IRON					
7 IRON					
6 IRON					
5 IRON					
4 IRON					
3 IRON					
HYBRID					
DRIVER					
CHIPPING					
PITCHING					
OUT OF BUNKER					
TOTAL					

FAVORITE MOMENTS _____
_____
_____

AREAS OF IMPROVEMENT _____
_____
_____

TOP 3 DRILLS TO PRACTICE

1 _____
2 _____
3 _____

PRACTICE LOG

START: _____ **END:** _____ S M T W T F S

CLUB/SHOT	DISTANCE GOAL	MINUTES PRACTICED	# OF BALLS	SHOTS MADE	SUCCESS RATIO
WARM UP					
PUTT					
PUTT					
PUTT					
PUTT					
9 IRON					
8 IRON					
7 IRON					
6 IRON					
5 IRON					
4 IRON					
3 IRON					
HYBRID					
DRIVER					
CHIPPING					
PITCHING					
OUT OF BUNKER					
TOTAL					

FAVORITE MOMENTS _____

_____

_____

AREAS OF IMPROVEMENT _____

_____

TOP 3 DRILLS TO PRACTICE

1 _____

2 _____

3 _____

GAME SCORE AND STATS

OVERVIEW: _____ **COURSE:** _____

DATE: _____ S M T W T F S

TOURNAMENT: YES ☐ NO ☐ **ROUND:** _____ **START:** _____ **END:** _____

EVENT NAME: _____ **TYPE:** 9 HOLES ☐ 18 HOLES ☐

WEATHER:

FRONT NINE	1	2	3	4	5	6	7	8	9	TOTAL
PAR										
FAIRWAYS HIT										
CLUB (TEE SHOT)										
GIR										
SUCCESSFUL SCRAMBLE										
PPR										
HANDICAP										
SCORE										

BACK NINE	10	11	12	13	14	15	16	17	18	TOTAL
PAR										
FAIRWAYS HIT										
CLUB (TEE SHOT)										
GIR										
SUCCESSFUL SCRAMBLE										
PPR										
HANDICAP										
SCORE										

NOTES: _____

TOTALS

REVIEW AND NOTES

SUMMARY

EAGLES:	BIRDIES:	PAR:
BOGEY:	DOUBLE BOGEY:	

TOTAL SCORE

REVIEW

TOTAL SCORE:	FAIRWAYS HIT:	DRIVING ACC %:
GIR %:	SCRAMBLE %:	AVERAGE PUTTS:

NOTES

COURSE CHALLENGES: _____

_____

_____

_____

_____

19TH HOLE: _____

_____

_____

_____

_____

RATE THE GREEN!

CONDITIONS: ○ ○ ○ ○ ○ ○ ○ ○ ○ ○

VALUE: ○ ○ ○ ○ ○ ○ ○ ○ ○ ○

LAYOUT: ○ ○ ○ ○ ○ ○ ○ ○ ○ ○

PACE OF PLAY: ○ ○ ○ ○ ○ ○ ○ ○ ○ ○

AMENITIES: ○ ○ ○ ○ ○ ○ ○ ○ ○ ○

OVERALL RATING: ____ / 100

GAME SCORE AND STATS

OVERVIEW: _____ **COURSE:** _____

DATE: _____ S M T W T F S

TOURNAMENT: YES ☐ NO ☐ **ROUND:** _____ **START:** _____ **END:** _____

EVENT NAME: _____ **TYPE:** 9 HOLES ☐ 18 HOLES ☐

WEATHER:

FRONT NINE	1	2	3	4	5	6	7	8	9	TOTAL
PAR										
FAIRWAYS HIT										
CLUB (TEE SHOT)										
GIR										
SUCCESSFUL SCRAMBLE										
PPR										
HANDICAP										
SCORE										

BACK NINE	10	11	12	13	14	15	16	17	18	TOTAL
PAR										
FAIRWAYS HIT										
CLUB (TEE SHOT)										
GIR										
SUCCESSFUL SCRAMBLE										
PPR										
HANDICAP										
SCORE										

NOTES: _____

TOTALS

REVIEW AND NOTES

SUMMARY		
EAGLES:	BIRDIES:	PAR:
BOGEY:	DOUBLE BOGEY:	

TOTAL SCORE

REVIEW		
TOTAL SCORE:	FAIRWAYS HIT:	DRIVING ACC %:
GIR %:	SCRAMBLE %:	AVERAGE PUTTS:

NOTES	
COURSE CHALLENGES: _____	19TH HOLE: _____

RATE THE GREEN!

CONDITIONS: ○ ○ ○ ○ ○ ○ ○ ○ ○ ○

VALUE: ○ ○ ○ ○ ○ ○ ○ ○ ○ ○

LAYOUT: ○ ○ ○ ○ ○ ○ ○ ○ ○ ○

PACE OF PLAY: ○ ○ ○ ○ ○ ○ ○ ○ ○ ○

AMENITIES: ○ ○ ○ ○ ○ ○ ○ ○ ○ ○

OVERALL RATING: ____ / 100

GAME SCORE AND STATS

OVERVIEW: _____ **COURSE:** _____

DATE: _____ S M T W T F S

TOURNAMENT: YES ☐ NO ☐ **ROUND:** _____ **START:** _____ **END:** _____

EVENT NAME: _____ **TYPE:** 9 HOLES ☐ 18 HOLES ☐

WEATHER:

FRONT NINE	1	2	3	4	5	6	7	8	9	TOTAL
PAR										
FAIRWAYS HIT										
CLUB (TEE SHOT)										
GIR										
SUCCESSFUL SCRAMBLE										
PPR										
HANDICAP										
SCORE										

BACK NINE	10	11	12	13	14	15	16	17	18	TOTAL
PAR										
FAIRWAYS HIT										
CLUB (TEE SHOT)										
GIR										
SUCCESSFUL SCRAMBLE										
PPR										
HANDICAP										
SCORE										

NOTES: _____

TOTALS

REVIEW AND NOTES

SUMMARY

EAGLES:	BIRDIES:	PAR:
BOGEY:	DOUBLE BOGEY:	

TOTAL SCORE

REVIEW

TOTAL SCORE:	FAIRWAYS HIT:	DRIVING ACC %:
GIR %:	SCRAMBLE %:	AVERAGE PUTTS:

NOTES

COURSE CHALLENGES: _____

_____
_____
_____
_____

19TH HOLE: _____

_____
_____
_____
_____

RATE THE GREEN!

CONDITIONS: ○ ○ ○ ○ ○ ○ ○ ○ ○ ○

VALUE: ○ ○ ○ ○ ○ ○ ○ ○ ○ ○

LAYOUT: ○ ○ ○ ○ ○ ○ ○ ○ ○ ○

PACE OF PLAY: ○ ○ ○ ○ ○ ○ ○ ○ ○ ○

AMENITIES: ○ ○ ○ ○ ○ ○ ○ ○ ○ ○

OVERALL RATING: ____ / 100

GAME SCORE AND STATS

OVERVIEW: _____ **COURSE:** _____

DATE: _____ S M T W T F S

TOURNAMENT: YES ☐ NO ☐ **ROUND:** _____ **START:** _____ **END:** _____

EVENT NAME: _____ **TYPE:** 9 HOLES ☐ 18 HOLES ☐

WEATHER:

FRONT NINE	1	2	3	4	5	6	7	8	9	TOTAL
PAR										
FAIRWAYS HIT										
CLUB (TEE SHOT)										
GIR										
SUCCESSFUL SCRAMBLE										
PPR										
HANDICAP										
SCORE										

BACK NINE	10	11	12	13	14	15	16	17	18	TOTAL
PAR										
FAIRWAYS HIT										
CLUB (TEE SHOT)										
GIR										
SUCCESSFUL SCRAMBLE										
PPR										
HANDICAP										
SCORE										

NOTES: _____

TOTALS

REVIEW AND NOTES

SUMMARY

EAGLES:	BIRDIES:	PAR:
BOGEY:	DOUBLE BOGEY:	

TOTAL SCORE

REVIEW

TOTAL SCORE:	FAIRWAYS HIT:	DRIVING ACC %:
GIR %:	SCRAMBLE %:	AVERAGE PUTTS:

NOTES

COURSE CHALLENGES: _____

_____

_____

_____

_____

19TH HOLE: _____

_____

_____

_____

_____

RATE THE GREEN!

CONDITIONS: ○ ○ ○ ○ ○ ○ ○ ○ ○ ○

VALUE: ○ ○ ○ ○ ○ ○ ○ ○ ○ ○

LAYOUT: ○ ○ ○ ○ ○ ○ ○ ○ ○ ○

PACE OF PLAY: ○ ○ ○ ○ ○ ○ ○ ○ ○ ○

AMENITIES: ○ ○ ○ ○ ○ ○ ○ ○ ○ ○

OVERALL RATING: ____ / 100

GAME SCORE AND STATS

OVERVIEW: _____ **COURSE:** _____

DATE: _____ S M T W T F S

TOURNAMENT: YES ☐ NO ☐ **ROUND:** _____ **START:** _____ **END:** _____

EVENT NAME: _____ **TYPE:** 9 HOLES ☐ 18 HOLES ☐

WEATHER:

FRONT NINE	1	2	3	4	5	6	7	8	9	TOTAL
PAR										
FAIRWAYS HIT										
CLUB (TEE SHOT)										
GIR										
SUCCESSFUL SCRAMBLE										
PPR										
HANDICAP										
SCORE										

BACK NINE	10	11	12	13	14	15	16	17	18	TOTAL
PAR										
FAIRWAYS HIT										
CLUB (TEE SHOT)										
GIR										
SUCCESSFUL SCRAMBLE										
PPR										
HANDICAP										
SCORE										

NOTES: _____

TOTALS

REVIEW AND NOTES

SUMMARY

| EAGLES: | BIRDIES: | PAR: |
| BOGEY: | DOUBLE BOGEY: | |

TOTAL SCORE

REVIEW

| TOTAL SCORE: | FAIRWAYS HIT: | DRIVING ACC %: |
| GIR %: | SCRAMBLE %: | AVERAGE PUTTS: |

NOTES

COURSE CHALLENGES: _____
_____
_____
_____
_____

19TH HOLE: _____
_____
_____
_____
_____

RATE THE GREEN!

CONDITIONS: ○ ○ ○ ○ ○ ○ ○ ○ ○ ○

VALUE: ○ ○ ○ ○ ○ ○ ○ ○ ○ ○

LAYOUT: ○ ○ ○ ○ ○ ○ ○ ○ ○ ○

PACE OF PLAY: ○ ○ ○ ○ ○ ○ ○ ○ ○ ○

AMENITIES: ○ ○ ○ ○ ○ ○ ○ ○ ○ ○

OVERALL RATING: _____ / 100

GAME SCORE AND STATS

OVERVIEW: _____ **COURSE:** _____

DATE: _____ S M T W T F S

TOURNAMENT: YES ☐ NO ☐ **ROUND:** _____ **START:** _____ **END:** _____

EVENT NAME: _____ **TYPE:** 9 HOLES ☐ 18 HOLES ☐

WEATHER:

FRONT NINE	1	2	3	4	5	6	7	8	9	TOTAL
PAR										
FAIRWAYS HIT										
CLUB (TEE SHOT)										
GIR										
SUCCESSFUL SCRAMBLE										
PPR										
HANDICAP										
SCORE										

BACK NINE	10	11	12	13	14	15	16	17	18	TOTAL
PAR										
FAIRWAYS HIT										
CLUB (TEE SHOT)										
GIR										
SUCCESSFUL SCRAMBLE										
PPR										
HANDICAP										
SCORE										

NOTES: _____
_____

TOTALS

REVIEW AND NOTES

SUMMARY		
EAGLES:	BIRDIES:	PAR:
BOGEY:	DOUBLE BOGEY:	

TOTAL SCORE

REVIEW		
TOTAL SCORE:	FAIRWAYS HIT:	DRIVING ACC %:
GIR %:	SCRAMBLE %:	AVERAGE PUTTS:

NOTES

COURSE CHALLENGES: _____

19TH HOLE: _____

RATE THE GREEN!

CONDITIONS: ○ ○ ○ ○ ○ ○ ○ ○ ○ ○ ○

VALUE: ○ ○ ○ ○ ○ ○ ○ ○ ○ ○ ○

LAYOUT: ○ ○ ○ ○ ○ ○ ○ ○ ○ ○ ○

PACE OF PLAY: ○ ○ ○ ○ ○ ○ ○ ○ ○ ○ ○

AMENITIES: ○ ○ ○ ○ ○ ○ ○ ○ ○ ○ ○

OVERALL RATING: ____ / 100

GAME SCORE AND STATS

OVERVIEW: _____ **COURSE:** _____

DATE: _____ S M T W T F S

TOURNAMENT: YES ☐ NO ☐ **ROUND:** _____ **START:** _____ **END:** _____

EVENT NAME: _____ **TYPE:** 9 HOLES ☐ 18 HOLES ☐

WEATHER:

FRONT NINE	1	2	3	4	5	6	7	8	9	TOTAL
PAR										
FAIRWAYS HIT										
CLUB (TEE SHOT)										
GIR										
SUCCESSFUL SCRAMBLE										
PPR										
HANDICAP										
SCORE										

BACK NINE	10	11	12	13	14	15	16	17	18	TOTAL
PAR										
FAIRWAYS HIT										
CLUB (TEE SHOT)										
GIR										
SUCCESSFUL SCRAMBLE										
PPR										
HANDICAP										
SCORE										

NOTES: _____

TOTALS

REVIEW AND NOTES

SUMMARY

EAGLES:	BIRDIES:	PAR:
BOGEY:	DOUBLE BOGEY:	

TOTAL SCORE

REVIEW

TOTAL SCORE:	FAIRWAYS HIT:	DRIVING ACC %:
GIR %:	SCRAMBLE %:	AVERAGE PUTTS:

NOTES

COURSE CHALLENGES: _____

19TH HOLE: _____

RATE THE GREEN!

CONDITIONS: ○ ○ ○ ○ ○ ○ ○ ○ ○ ○

VALUE: ○ ○ ○ ○ ○ ○ ○ ○ ○ ○

LAYOUT: ○ ○ ○ ○ ○ ○ ○ ○ ○ ○

PACE OF PLAY: ○ ○ ○ ○ ○ ○ ○ ○ ○ ○

AMENITIES: ○ ○ ○ ○ ○ ○ ○ ○ ○ ○

OVERALL RATING: ____ / 100

GAME SCORE AND STATS

OVERVIEW: _____ **COURSE:** _____

DATE: _____ S M T W T F S

TOURNAMENT: YES ☐ NO ☐ **ROUND:** _____ **START:** _____ **END:** _____

EVENT NAME: _____ **TYPE:** 9 HOLES ☐ 18 HOLES ☐

WEATHER:

FRONT NINE	1	2	3	4	5	6	7	8	9	TOTAL
PAR										
FAIRWAYS HIT										
CLUB (TEE SHOT)										
GIR										
SUCCESSFUL SCRAMBLE										
PPR										
HANDICAP										
SCORE										

BACK NINE	10	11	12	13	14	15	16	17	18	TOTAL
PAR										
FAIRWAYS HIT										
CLUB (TEE SHOT)										
GIR										
SUCCESSFUL SCRAMBLE										
PPR										
HANDICAP										
SCORE										

NOTES: _____

TOTALS

REVIEW AND NOTES

SUMMARY		
EAGLES:	BIRDIES:	PAR:
BOGEY:	DOUBLE BOGEY:	

TOTAL SCORE

REVIEW		
TOTAL SCORE:	FAIRWAYS HIT:	DRIVING ACC %:
GIR %:	SCRAMBLE %:	AVERAGE PUTTS:

NOTES

COURSE CHALLENGES: _____

_____
_____
_____
_____
_____

19TH HOLE: _____

_____
_____
_____
_____
_____

RATE THE GREEN!

CONDITIONS: ○ ○ ○ ○ ○ ○ ○ ○ ○ ○

VALUE: ○ ○ ○ ○ ○ ○ ○ ○ ○ ○

LAYOUT: ○ ○ ○ ○ ○ ○ ○ ○ ○ ○

PACE OF PLAY: ○ ○ ○ ○ ○ ○ ○ ○ ○ ○

AMENITIES: ○ ○ ○ ○ ○ ○ ○ ○ ○ ○

OVERALL RATING: ____ / 100

GAME SCORE AND STATS

OVERVIEW: _____ **COURSE:** _____

DATE: _____ S M T W T F S

TOURNAMENT: YES ☐ NO ☐ **ROUND:** _____ **START:** _____ **END:** _____

EVENT NAME: _____ **TYPE:** 9 HOLES ☐ 18 HOLES ☐

WEATHER:

FRONT NINE	1	2	3	4	5	6	7	8	9	TOTAL
PAR										
FAIRWAYS HIT										
CLUB (TEE SHOT)										
GIR										
SUCCESSFUL SCRAMBLE										
PPR										
HANDICAP										
SCORE										

BACK NINE	10	11	12	13	14	15	16	17	18	TOTAL
PAR										
FAIRWAYS HIT										
CLUB (TEE SHOT)										
GIR										
SUCCESSFUL SCRAMBLE										
PPR										
HANDICAP										
SCORE										

NOTES: _____

TOTALS

REVIEW AND NOTES

SUMMARY

EAGLES:	BIRDIES:	PAR:
BOGEY:	DOUBLE BOGEY:	

TOTAL SCORE

REVIEW

TOTAL SCORE:	FAIRWAYS HIT:	DRIVING ACC %:
GIR %:	SCRAMBLE %:	AVERAGE PUTTS:

NOTES

COURSE CHALLENGES: _____

19TH HOLE: _____

RATE THE GREEN!

CONDITIONS: ○ ○ ○ ○ ○ ○ ○ ○ ○ ○

VALUE: ○ ○ ○ ○ ○ ○ ○ ○ ○ ○

LAYOUT: ○ ○ ○ ○ ○ ○ ○ ○ ○ ○

PACE OF PLAY: ○ ○ ○ ○ ○ ○ ○ ○ ○ ○

AMENITIES: ○ ○ ○ ○ ○ ○ ○ ○ ○ ○

OVERALL RATING: ____ / 100

GAME SCORE AND STATS

OVERVIEW: _____ **COURSE:** _____

DATE: _____ S M T W T F S

TOURNAMENT: YES ☐ NO ☐ **ROUND:** _____ **START:** _____ **END:** _____

EVENT NAME: _____ **TYPE:** 9 HOLES ☐ 18 HOLES ☐

WEATHER:

FRONT NINE	1	2	3	4	5	6	7	8	9	TOTAL
PAR										
FAIRWAYS HIT										
CLUB (TEE SHOT)										
GIR										
SUCCESSFUL SCRAMBLE										
PPR										
HANDICAP										
SCORE										

BACK NINE	10	11	12	13	14	15	16	17	18	TOTAL
PAR										
FAIRWAYS HIT										
CLUB (TEE SHOT)										
GIR										
SUCCESSFUL SCRAMBLE										
PPR										
HANDICAP										
SCORE										

NOTES: _____

TOTALS

REVIEW AND NOTES

SUMMARY

| EAGLES: | BIRDIES: | PAR: |
| BOGEY: | DOUBLE BOGEY: | |

TOTAL SCORE

REVIEW

| TOTAL SCORE: | FAIRWAYS HIT: | DRIVING ACC %: |
| GIR %: | SCRAMBLE %: | AVERAGE PUTTS: |

NOTES

COURSE CHALLENGES: _____
_____
_____
_____
_____

19TH HOLE: _____
_____
_____
_____
_____

RATE THE GREEN!

CONDITIONS: ◯ ◯ ◯ ◯ ◯ ◯ ◯ ◯ ◯ ◯

VALUE: ◯ ◯ ◯ ◯ ◯ ◯ ◯ ◯ ◯ ◯

LAYOUT: ◯ ◯ ◯ ◯ ◯ ◯ ◯ ◯ ◯ ◯

PACE OF PLAY: ◯ ◯ ◯ ◯ ◯ ◯ ◯ ◯ ◯ ◯

AMENITIES: ◯ ◯ ◯ ◯ ◯ ◯ ◯ ◯ ◯ ◯

OVERALL RATING: ____ / 100

GAME SCORE AND STATS

OVERVIEW: _____ **COURSE:** _____

DATE: _____ S M T W T F S

TOURNAMENT: YES ☐ NO ☐ **ROUND:** _____ **START:** _____ **END:** _____

EVENT NAME: _____ **TYPE:** 9 HOLES ☐ 18 HOLES ☐

WEATHER: ☀ ⛅ ☁ 🌦 ❄ ⛈

FRONT NINE	1	2	3	4	5	6	7	8	9	TOTAL
PAR										
FAIRWAYS HIT										
CLUB (TEE SHOT)										
GIR										
SUCCESSFUL SCRAMBLE										
PPR										
HANDICAP										
SCORE										

BACK NINE	10	11	12	13	14	15	16	17	18	TOTAL
PAR										
FAIRWAYS HIT										
CLUB (TEE SHOT)										
GIR										
SUCCESSFUL SCRAMBLE										
PPR										
HANDICAP										
SCORE										

NOTES: _____

TOTALS

REVIEW AND NOTES

SUMMARY		
EAGLES:	BIRDIES:	PAR:
BOGEY:	DOUBLE BOGEY:	

TOTAL SCORE

REVIEW		
TOTAL SCORE:	FAIRWAYS HIT:	DRIVING ACC %:
GIR %:	SCRAMBLE %:	AVERAGE PUTTS:

NOTES	
COURSE CHALLENGES: _____	19TH HOLE: _____

RATE THE GREEN!

CONDITIONS: ○ ○ ○ ○ ○ ○ ○ ○ ○ ○ ○

VALUE: ○ ○ ○ ○ ○ ○ ○ ○ ○ ○ ○

LAYOUT: ○ ○ ○ ○ ○ ○ ○ ○ ○ ○ ○

PACE OF PLAY: ○ ○ ○ ○ ○ ○ ○ ○ ○ ○ ○

AMENITIES: ○ ○ ○ ○ ○ ○ ○ ○ ○ ○ ○

OVERALL RATING: ____ / 100

CALENDAR

RECORD THE DAYS YOU'VE PRACTICED OR PLAYED

MONTH: _____ YEAR: _____

S	M	T	W	T	F	S

MONTH: _____ **YEAR:** _____

S	M	T	W	T	F	S

CALENDAR

RECORD THE DAYS YOU'VE PRACTICED OR PLAYED

MONTH:				YEAR:		
S	M	T	W	T	F	S

MONTH: _____ **YEAR:** _____

S	M	T	W	T	F	S

CALENDAR

RECORD THE DAYS YOU'VE PRACTICED OR PLAYED

MONTH:				YEAR:	
S	M	T	W	T	F	S

MONTH: _____ **YEAR:** _____

S	M	T	W	T	F	S

CALENDAR

RECORD THE DAYS YOU'VE PRACTICED OR PLAYED

MONTH: _____ **YEAR:** _____

S	M	T	W	T	F	S

MONTH: _____ **YEAR:** _____

S	M	T	W	T	F	S

CALENDAR

RECORD THE DAYS YOU'VE PRACTICED OR PLAYED

MONTH:				YEAR:		
S	M	T	W	T	F	S

MONTH: _____ **YEAR:** _____

S	M	T	W	T	F	S

CALENDAR

RECORD THE DAYS YOU'VE PRACTICED OR PLAYED

MONTH: _____ YEAR: _____

S	M	T	W	T	F	S

MONTH: _____ **YEAR:** _____

S	M	T	W	T	F	S

© 2025 by Quarto Publishing Group USA Inc.

First published in 2025 by Rock Point,
an imprint of The Quarto Group,
142 West 36th Street, 4th Floor,
New York, NY 10018, USA
(212) 779-4972 www.Quarto.com

All rights reserved. No part of this book may be reproduced in any form without written permission of the copyright owners. All images in this book have been reproduced with the knowledge and prior consent of the artists concerned, and no responsibility is accepted by producer, publisher, or printer for any infringement of copyright or otherwise, arising from the contents of this publication. Every effort has been made to ensure that credits accurately comply with information supplied. We apologize for any inaccuracies that may have occurred and will resolve inaccurate or missing information in a subsequent reprinting of the book.

Rock Point titles are also available at discount for retail, wholesale, promotional, and bulk purchase. For details, contact the Special Sales Manager by email at specialsales@quarto.com or by mail at The Quarto Group, Attn: Special Sales Manager, 100 Cummings Center Suite 265D, Beverly, MA 01915 USA.

10 9 8 7 6 5 4 3 2 1

ISBN: 978-1-57715-487-7

Group Publisher: Rage Kindelsperger
Editorial Director: Erin Canning
Creative Director: Laura Drew
Managing Editor: Cara Donaldson
Editorial Assistants: Tobiah Agurkis and Alyana Nurani
Cover and Interior Design: Kegley Design

Printed in China